THE VEGAN ATHLETE:

A REVOLUTIONARY APPROACH TO CLIMAX PERFORMANCE

BY

ELLA RICE

Copyright © by Ella Rice 2023. All rights reserved.

Before this document is duplicated or reproduced in any manner, the publisher's consent must be gained.

Therefore, the contents within can never be stored electronically, transferred, or kept in a database. Neither in part nor in full can the document be copied, scanned, faxed, or retained without approval from the publisher or creator.

Table of Contents

Introduction

In recent years, there has been a remarkable shift in the world of athletics and fitness. A growing number of athletes, from amateurs to professionals, are embracing a plant-based lifestyle and achieving extraordinary feats of strength, endurance, and overall performance. "The Vegan Athlete: A Revolutionary Approach to Climax Performance" is a groundbreaking book that explores the transformative power of plant-based nutrition and its profound impact on athletic abilities.

This book aims to challenge the prevailing belief that animal products are essential for peak athletic performance. It delves deep into the science behind plant-based nutrition, unveiling the many ways it can optimize performance, enhance recovery, and unlock the full potential of athletes. Whether you are a seasoned competitor, a recreational athlete, or someone seeking to improve their fitness levels, this book presents an innovative approach to achieving peak performance while upholding ethical and environmental values.

Chapter 1

Understanding The Power Behind The Food: Macronutrients, Micronutrients, And Calorie Density

In the contemporary world, food has evolved from only being a source of nourishment to a dynamic and complicated field of study. The power of food comes from its capacity to fuel our bodies and have an effect on our general health and well-being. The important constituents that makeup food, including macronutrients, micronutrients, and calorie density, will be discussed in this chapter. By grasping these ideas, you'll be better equipped to choose your meals wisely and maximize your nutrient intake.

Macronutrients:

The main nutrients in our diet that provide us with energy and are necessary for our bodies' development are known as macronutrients. Carbohydrates, proteins, and lipids are among them. Every macronutrient contributes differently to our general wellness.

1. Carbohydrates: Our bodies get their energy primarily from carbohydrates. Foods like grains,

fruits, vegetables, and legumes contain them. Simple and complex carbs are additional categories for categorizing carbohydrates. Simple carbs, such as those in processed sweets and sugary drinks, are easily absorbed and provide you with a quick but fleeting energy boost. Whole grains and starchy vegetables contain complex carbohydrates that are metabolized more gradually and offer sustained energy and crucial fiber.

2. Proteins: Proteins are essential for the development, maintenance, and repair of the tissues in our bodies. They are made up of amino acids, which serve as the foundation for

proteins. Meat, poultry, fish, eggs, dairy products, legumes, and nuts are all excellent sources of protein. We can be sure we're getting all the essential amino acids our bodies need by consuming a range of protein sources.

3. Fats: Fats are necessary for a number of body processes, including the production of energy, the insulation of organs, and the absorption of vitamins that are fat-soluble. Avocados, nuts, seeds, fatty seafood, and plant oils are all good sources of healthy fat. Monounsaturated and polyunsaturated fats are good sources of unsaturated fats; select them over

saturated and trans fats, which can cause heart disease.

Micronutrients:

The energy and fundamental building blocks are provided by macronutrients, whereas vitamins, minerals, and trace elements, which are needed in lower amounts but are crucial for many physiological processes, are known as micronutrients.

1. Vitamins: Vitamins are organic substances required for a number of bodily functions. They help enzymes carry out crucial processes by acting as cofactors and coenzymes. Vitamins

can either be fat-soluble (like vitamins A, D, E, and K) or water-soluble (like vitamins B and C). Each vitamin plays a unique part in promoting energy production, bone health, immunological function, and a variety of other processes.

2. Minerals: Minerals are inorganic substances that are essential for preserving fluid equilibrium and biological functioning. They contribute to the development of hormones and enzymes, muscular contraction, bone health, and nerve and enzyme creation. Calcium, iron, zinc, magnesium, and potassium are a few minerals. An appropriate intake of important minerals can be made

possible by consuming a varied diet that features a variety of fruits, vegetables, whole grains, and nuts.

Energy Density:

The quantity of calories in a specific volume or weight of food is referred to as the calorie density. Making healthy eating choices and managing weight might be aided by understanding calorie density.

1. Foods that are low in calories per unit of volume are known as low-calorie-dense foods. Generally speaking, foods like fruits, vegetables, whole grains, and legumes are low in calories but high

in fiber and other nutrients. These foods can support satiety and offer crucial nutrients, minerals and vitamins while keeping a healthy weight.

2. Foods that are high in calories per serving: Foods that are high in calories per serving include processed foods, fried foods, and sugary snacks. Regular use of these foods can lead to weight gain and raise your chance of developing chronic diseases. It's crucial to pay attention to portion sizes and give high-nutrient, low-calorie foods priority.

A thorough understanding of macronutrients, micronutrients, and calorie density is necessary to grasp the power of food. You may maximize your nutritional intake and promote your general health by implementing a balanced diet that consists of a mix of whole foods rich in macronutrients and micronutrients while taking calorie density into account. Keep in mind that food serves as both a fuel source and a way to nurture your body and improve your well-being.

Chapter 2

It's time to have the protein talk

One important element frequently takes center stage in our quest to understand nutrition and sustain a healthy lifestyle: protein. The importance of the macronutrient protein to our overall health cannot be overstated. Protein is a vital component of our diet because it helps us create and repair tissues, maintain immunological health, and provide energy. However, despite its significance, protein is still poorly understood by many people, who also struggle to successfully incorporate it into their daily lives. We will go into the realm of protein in this chapter, talking about its uses, sources, and how crucial it is to have the "protein talk" in order to maximize our dietary intake.

Protein: The Foundation of Life

Proteins are substantial, intricate molecules made of amino acids. These amino acids serve as the building blocks for the synthesis and upkeep of tissues in our body, including muscles, skin, hair, and organs. Proteins play crucial roles in a variety of metabolic processes and immunological responses in addition to their structural function. Proteins also function as enzymes, hormones, and antibodies.

Learning About Protein Needs

Age, sex, activity level, and overall objectives all play a role in determining the proper protein intake for good health. Adults are advised to ingest 0.8 grams of protein per kilogram of body weight per day, according to the Recommended Dietary Allowance (RDA). This recommendation might not, however, apply to everyone. In order to assist muscle repair and recovery, athletes, those undergoing severe physical training, and people with certain medical disorders may need to consume more protein.

Protein Resources

Protein can be found in both plant and animal sources. Meat, poultry, fish, eggs, and dairy products are examples of animal-based protein sources that are considered complete proteins because they include all the essential amino acids that our bodies need. Legumes, nuts, seeds, grains, and some vegetables are all sources of plant-based protein, but they are typically incomplete proteins because they lack one or more important amino acids. But one can get a full protein profile by combining several plant-based protein sources, like beans and rice or hummus and pita bread.

Protein quality and digestibility

A protein's nutritional value is mostly dependent on its quality and digestion in addition to its quantity. The presence and proportion of necessary amino acids determine the concept of protein quality. Proteins derived from animals often have higher biological value and sufficient levels of all necessary amino acids. However, when mixed appropriately to preserve amino acid balance, plant-based proteins can still be very nutrient-dense. The term "digestibility" describes the body's capacity to digest and assimilate protein. Although plant-based proteins can be made more digestible through cooking and other food preparation techniques, animal-based proteins are often easier to digest than plant-based proteins.

Improved Protein Intake

Quantity and quality of protein consumption must be taken into account in order to maximize it. Higher protein intake throughout the day may be advantageous for anyone looking to increase or maintain muscle mass, such as athletes or senior citizens. It can also help to appropriately distribute your protein consumption throughout the day. Various protein sources, both animal and plant-based, can be combined to provide a wide range of amino acid profiles. A balanced diet can also be maintained by including lean sources of protein and limiting additional carbohydrates and fats.

Correcting Illusions and Concerns

Numerous myths about consuming enough protein have surfaced in recent years. Some people are concerned that eating too much protein could have negative health repercussions, like kidney damage or osteoporosis. However, high-protein diets are typically safe for healthy people. It is crucial to remember that those with pre-existing kidney issues should speak with their doctor for specific suggestions. Additionally, as long as great attention is taken to balancing amino acid consumption, plant-based proteins can sufficiently provide protein requirements for people following vegetarian or vegan diets.

A healthy diet must include protein because it is a necessary building block for the development and operation of our bodies. By comprehending the roles, sources, and significance of protein, we may have the "protein talk" to maximize our dietary intake. A well-rounded and nourishing diet can be attained by balancing protein amount and quality, including a range of protein sources, and debunking myths about protein intake. In order to enhance our general health and well-being, we might prioritize protein in our daily life.

Chapter 3

Carbohydrates: the body's perfect fuel

In our diet, carbohydrates are essential because they are the body's preferred source of energy. These macronutrients are a varied category that can be found in a variety of foods, such as cereals, fruits, vegetables, and dairy products. We will delve into the numerous forms, uses, and effects of carbs on general health and performance as well as its significance as a fuel source for the body in this chapter.

1. Getting to Know Carbohydrates:

Carbon, hydrogen, and oxygen atoms make up the chemical molecules known as carbohydrates. Sugars, carbohydrates, and dietary fiber are the three basic categories into which they fall. Simple carbohydrates like glucose and fructose are sugars that give the body instant energy. Starches are complex carbohydrates that are digested into glucose and can be found in foods like potatoes and grains. Dietary fiber, which is found in fruits, vegetables, and whole grains, has many health advantages, such as better digestion and blood sugar control.

2. The Function of Carbohydrates in the Production of Energy

The body uses carbohydrates as its main fuel source. They are converted into glucose after consumption, which travels to all of the body's cells via the bloodstream. The liver and muscles can store glucose as glycogen for later use or utilize it right away for energy. Glycogen stores are drawn upon to maintain energy levels during intervals of vigorous physical exercise or protracted fasting.

3. Nutritional intake and athletic performance:

Exercise performance is significantly impacted by carbohydrates. A sufficient intake of carbohydrates can increase endurance, postpone exhaustion, and speed up recovery during and after physical activity. The body heavily relies on its glycogen reserves for sustenance during high-intensity exercise. Prior to exercise, taking carbs maintains adequate glycogen levels, while consuming them while exercising can give working muscles a consistent supply of glucose. Consuming carbohydrates after exercise aids in replenishing glycogen reserves and accelerates the healing process.

4. Carbohydrates and Mental Performance:

The main source of energy for the brain is glucose, which is derived from carbs. About 20% of the body's total energy is expended by the brain, which needs a steady supply of glucose to operate at its best. Inadequate carbohydrate intake can cause memory loss, trouble concentrating, and a decline in cognitive function. A continuous supply of glucose to the brain is ensured by including complex carbohydrates in the diet, such as whole grains and fruits, enhancing mental performance.

5. Controlling Intake of Carbohydrates:

Although the body needs carbohydrates to function, it's crucial to consume them in moderation. A diet high in carbs, especially refined grains, and simple sugars, can raise the risk of developing insulin resistance, weight gain, and chronic illnesses including diabetes and heart disease. On the other side, significantly limiting carbohydrate intake might result in dietary deficits, low energy levels, and subpar athletic performance.

6. Picking Healthy Sources of Carbohydrates:

For optimal health and well-being, choose complete food sources of carbs that are high in nutrients. Along with carbohydrates, whole grains, legumes, fruits, and vegetables offer a variety of vitamins, minerals, and dietary fiber. These foods assist healthy digestion, encourage satiety, and provide long-lasting energy. Contrarily, processed meals like white bread, drinks, and sugary snacks offer empty calories and are deficient in important nutrients.

The body uses carbohydrates as its ideal fuel to power both physical and mental activity. Making dietary decisions based on knowledge of how carbs affect energy production, exercise performance, and cognitive function. We can provide a consistent source of energy while keeping excellent health by putting a priority on whole meals and complex carbs. It's crucial to strike a balance between the body's energy requirements and general well-being when it comes to carbohydrate intake.

Chapter 4

Recover better, train more

The primary focus of the fitness and sports industries is frequent training. The crucial role that recovery plays in enhancing performance and attaining long-term success is something that many athletes and fitness enthusiasts overlook. In this chapter, we'll examine the value of recuperation, talk about efficient recovery techniques, and discover how to balance training and rest for improved performance.

1. Recognizing the Value of Recovery:

a)   Recovery's   Function   in Performance:

Recovery is the process by which the body heals and acclimates to the strain that training places on it. It enables the replenishment of energy reserves, the restoration of harmed tissues, and the consolidation of knowledge and skill acquisition. For injury   avoidance,   avoiding overtraining,   and   maximizing performance gains, proper recuperation is essential.

b) The Impact of Overtraining:

When a person pushes their body beyond its capacity to recuperate from training stress, overtraining results. Performance suffers, injury risk rises, hormonal imbalances, mood swings, and immune system suppression occur as a result. Long-term success depends on recognizing the symptoms of overtraining and placing a high priority on recovery.

2. The Elements of Successful Recovery

a) Sleep and rest:

Recovery requires plenty of sleep. It enables the body to restore hormonal equilibrium, replenish energy reserves, and repair and rebuild damaged tissues. Since it improves immune system performance, memory consolidation, and muscular rehabilitation, quality sleep is particularly crucial. Sleep for 7-9 hours each night, undisturbed.

b) Hydration and Food:

The right kind of nourishment is essential for recuperation. A balanced diet that includes enough protein, carbs, and healthy fats gives the body the building blocks it needs to repair tissues and restores energy reserves. Water is involved in many physiological processes, therefore staying hydrated is essential for a speedy recovery.

c) Active Recovery

Low-intensity exercises, such as light aerobics or easy stretching, help speed up the healing process by increasing blood flow, easing tightness in the muscles, and assisting in the clearance of metabolic waste products. Additionally, active recuperation might improve psychological health and encourage relaxation.

d) Bodywork & Massage:

Muscle tension can be reduced, flexibility can be improved, and circulation can be improved through massage and other bodywork techniques like foam rolling and stretching. These methods encourage endorphin release, lessen inflammation, and hasten the healing process.

3. Mind-Body Recovery Methods:

a) Mindfulness and meditation

Utilizing mindfulness techniques, such as deep breathing exercises or meditation, can help reduce stress, increase concentration, and encourage mental calm. These methods help general healing by lowering anxiety, improving sleep quality, and decreasing insomnia.

b) Stretching and yoga:

Yoga offers a thorough approach to recovery by incorporating physical postures, breathing techniques, and mindfulness. It boosts body awareness, promotes relaxation, balances strength, and increases flexibility, which helps recovery and prevents injuries.

4. Assessing and modifying the training load:

a) Pay Attention to Your Body:

For the purpose of avoiding overtraining and maximizing recovery, it is essential to pay attention to your body's signals and adapt training intensity and volume properly. Recognize the symptoms of tiredness, a lack of motivation, or prolonged muscular soreness and adjust your training program as appropriate.

b) Deloading and periodization

Periodization, an organized training cycle, enables scheduled intervals of decreased volume and intensity. Deloading weeks or microcycles provide the body more time to recover, preventing plateaus, lowering injury risk, and improving long-term performance.

Any training program must include recovery as a key component. Athletes and fitness enthusiasts can improve performance, avoid injuries, and achieve long-term success by prioritizing and putting efficient recuperation practices into practice. It's important to keep in mind that improving your recovery will help you train more successfully and efficiently.

Chapter 5

Unleashing your inner athlete

Athleticism is not just for elite athletes or those with special genetic abilities. Each of us has the capacity to awaken our inner athletes and access a world of strength on both the physical and mental levels. In this chapter, we'll look at the tactics, frame of mind, and training methods that will help you tap into your inner athlete so you can perform at your best and accomplish your athletic goals. Whether you're a novice or an experienced athlete, the ideas presented here will give you the confidence you need to overcome obstacles, go beyond your potential, and improve.

1. Fostering an athlete's mentality:

It's crucial to develop an athlete's mindset before starting your athletic career. Discipline, tenacity, resiliency, and confidence in your own skills are all parts of this approach. The following are important guidelines to follow:

a) Setting goals: Clearly state your sports objectives and divide them into more manageable, short-term objectives. This will offer you a feeling of direction and purpose, which will keep you inspired throughout your journey.

b) Positive Self-Talk: Use positive affirmations to replace negative ideas and self-doubt. Create a powerful inner dialogue that supports and inspires you, strengthening your faith in your talents.

c) Accepting Failure: Recognize that failure is a prerequisite for success. Learn from failures, modify your strategy, and seize the chance to advance.

d) Mental imagery: Picture yourself achieving your sports goals. To maintain a positive outlook, visualize every aspect of your preparation, competition, and victory.

2. Creating a Stable Foundation:

Establishing a solid base of physical fitness and general well-being is necessary before you can unleash your inner athlete. This foundation combines flexibility, weight training, cardiovascular endurance, and good nutrition. Here is how to get going:

a) Engage in aerobic exercises like cycling, swimming, dancing, or jogging to increase your cardiovascular endurance. To improve your cardiovascular fitness, gradually increase the length and intensity of your workouts.

b) Strength training: Include resistance exercises in your regimen to improve your physical endurance, strength, and power. Pay attention to compound exercises like squats, deadlifts, bench presses, and pull-ups because they work in several muscular groups.

c) Flexibility and Mobility: Mobility exercises and stretching increase your range of motion, lower your risk of injury, and improve athletic performance. Your pre-and post-workout routines should include both static and dynamic stretches.

d) Nutrition and Hydration: Give your body the fuel it needs by eating a diet that is well-balanced and rich in lean proteins, complex carbs, healthy fats, and a variety of fruits and vegetables. Drink plenty of water all day long, especially when exercising.

3. Developing Sports-Related Skills:

Focusing on building sport-specific skills is essential if you want to unlock your inner athlete. Making improvements in your chosen sport-related skills will speed up your training, whether you're learning martial arts, playing soccer, or running a marathon. The following are some crucial tactics:

a) Technical training: Learn proper skills, form, and mechanics with the help of a coach or instructor. Break up complicated moves into smaller parts, and perfect each one before moving on to the next.

b) Exercises that mimic the movements and demands of your

sport should be incorporated into functional training (b). Your balance, agility, coordination, and proprioception will all improve as a result.

c) Mental conditioning: Increase mental toughness by engaging in mindfulness, meditation, and visualization exercises. Develop the ability to maintain attention under duress and to ignore outside distractions.

d) Sports-Specific Drills: Include exercises and simulations that reflect game or competition situations. Your capacity for judgment, quickness of response, and situational awareness will all improve as a result.

Adopting a Holistic Approach

Adopting a holistic strategy that considers your physical, mental, and emotional well-being is crucial if you want to completely unlock your inner athlete. Please take into account:

a) Rest and recovery are important. Give your body enough time to recuperate and adjust to the demands of exercise. Include rest days in your calendar, place a high priority on getting enough sleep, and use active recovery techniques like foam rolling and light stretching.

b) Injury Prevention: Prevent injuries by being proactive and paying attention to your body. You should also avoid overtraining and include injury-prevention exercises in your daily routine. Each workout should begin with a suitable warm-up and end with a cool-down.

c) Mental and Emotional Support: Look for a network of mentors, team members, or training partners who can offer direction, inspiration, and encouragement. To build mental toughness and manage stress caused by performance, think about working with a sports psychologist.

d) Maintain a healthy balance between your sports endeavors and other facets of your life. Maintain positive connections, engage in activities aside from sports, and give yourself time to unwind and recharge.

It takes commitment, self-control, and a growth mentality to unleash your inner athlete on this transforming journey. You may reach your full athletic potential by developing an athlete's mentality, establishing a strong physical foundation, learning sport-specific skills, and adopting a holistic approach. Keep in mind that growth requires patience, hard work, and persistence. With each step you go forward, you will have a better grasp of who you are and what you are capable of. Accept the process, have faith in your abilities, and let your competitive side come out.

Chapter 6

A Day in the Life of a plant-based athlete

More athletes are relying on plant-based diets to support their performance and advance general health and well-being in recent years. Numerous advantages of switching to a plant-based diet include accelerated physical recovery, more energy, and less inflammation. We will examine a typical day in the life of a plant-based athlete in this chapter, from sunrise to night, emphasizing the important ideas and tactics for maximizing diet, exercise, and recuperation.

1. Daily Schedule:

The day's tone is established in the morning. How a vegan athlete might begin their day is as follows:

a) After a night of sleep, start by hydrating your body with a big glass of water. For additional health advantages, add a squeeze of lemon or a dash of apple cider vinegar.

b) Breakfast: Start the day off right with a nutrient-rich, plant-based meal. Consider choices like an overnight oats bowl with nuts, seeds, and berries on top, or a smoothie made with fruit, leafy greens, and plant-based protein powder.

c) Supplementation: Give important vitamins like vitamin B12, vitamin D, and omega-3 fatty acids some thought for including in your morning routine. To find the supplements that are best for you, speak with a qualified nutritionist or member of the medical profession.

2. Performance and Training:

The main goals of a plant-based athlete's training regimen are performance and recuperation enhancement. A typical training session might go like this:

a) Pre-Workout Fuel: Eat a quick-to-digest snack between 30 and 60 minutes prior to the activity. A banana with almond butter, a handful of nuts, or a handmade energy bar with dates and nuts are all possible options.

b) Hydration: Drink plenty of water or a plant-based electrolyte drink throughout your workout to be properly hydrated. A natural sweetener like maple syrup can be combined with water, lemon juice, a teaspoon of sea salt, and other ingredients to create your own.

c) Post-Workout Refueling: After a workout, replenish your body with a mix of carbohydrates and plant-based protein. This may be a smoothie made with fruits, a plant-based protein powder, and a source of good fats like flaxseed or nut butter as a post-workout treat.

3. Improving the Nutrition from Plants:

For their nutritional needs, plant-based athletes give priority to entire, nutrient-dense diets. Here are some important guidelines to bear in mind:

a) Macronutrients: Make sure you get enough carbs, protein, and fat. Whole grains, fruits, and vegetables are among the sources of plant-based carbohydrates. Legumes, tofu, tempeh, seitan, and plant-based protein powders are examples of sources of plant-based protein. Nuts, seeds, avocados, and plant-based oils all include healthy fats.

b) Micronutrients: Pay close attention to important micronutrients, such as vitamin B12, iron, calcium, and omega-3 fatty acids, which are frequently included in animal products. These can be gained by consuming fortified foods or by including plant-based sources such as nutritional yeast, leafy greens, legumes, fortified plant-based milk, flaxseeds, or chia seeds.

c) Variety and Color: Include a wide range of plant-based foods in your diet to ensure that you are getting a variety of vitamins, minerals, and phytonutrients. On your plate, try to include a variety of colorful fruits, vegetables, whole grains, beans, nuts, and seeds.

d) Meal Preparation and Planning: Make sure you have a variety of healthy, plant-based meals on hand by planning your meals in advance. Set aside time each week for meal preparation to streamline the procedure and increase accessibility to healthier options.

4. Rest and Recovery:

For a plant-based athlete's general health and performance, proper recuperation and rest are crucial. Think about the following tactics:

a) In order to assist muscle rehabilitation and refuel energy reserves, continue to prioritize nutrient-dense, plant-based meals, and snacks throughout the day. Mix in a variety of healthful fats, proteins, and carbohydrates.

b) Quality sleep should be prioritized in order to enhance recovery and hormone regulation. Establish a regular sleep schedule and aim for 7-9 hours of sound sleep each night.

c) Active recuperation: To encourage blood flow, mobility, and recuperation on rest days, take part in low-impact exercises like gentle stretching, yoga, or mild aerobic exercise.

d) Mindfulness and Stress Reduction: Use mindfulness techniques to reduce stress and support mental health, such as journaling, deep breathing exercises, and meditation.

A plant-based athlete's day is dedicated to maximizing diet, exercise, and recovery to support both general health and athletic performance. Plant-based athletes can reach their maximum potential by putting an emphasis on complete diets made from plants, drinking plenty of water, and adopting a balanced approach to training and recovery. Remember that every person is different, so it's crucial to pay attention to your body's demands and get advice from a medical practitioner or qualified dietitian to make sure you're fulfilling your particular nutritional needs. Discover the remarkable advantages of a plant-based lifestyle for athletic success and well-being by embracing the power of plants.

www.ingramcontent.com/pod-product-compliance
Lightning Source LLC
Chambersburg PA
CBHW051847250726
48659CB00006B/2070